MENTAL HEALTH NURSING
Practical Record Book
for General Nursing and Midwifery

Mental Health Nursing Practical Record Book for General Nursing and Midwifery

R Sreevani
PhD in Psychiatric Nursing
Professor and Head
Department of Psychiatric Nursing
Dharwad Institute of Mental Health and Neurosciences (DIMHANS)
Dharwad, Karnataka, India

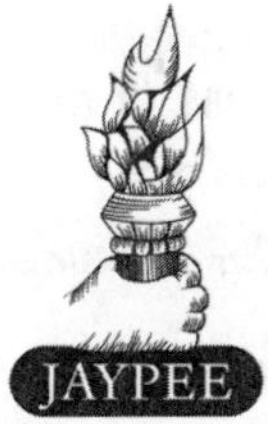

JAYPEE BROTHERS MEDICAL PUBLISHERS
The Health Sciences Publisher
New Delhi | London

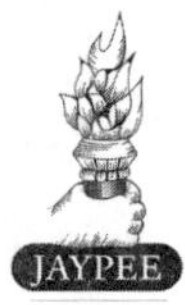

Jaypee Brothers Medical Publishers (P) Ltd

Headquarters
EMCA House
23/23-B, Ansari Road, Daryaganj
New Delhi 110 002, India
Landline: +91-11-23272143, +91-11-23272703
+91-11-23282021, +91-11-23245672
E-mail: jaypee@jaypeebrothers.com

Corporate Office
Jaypee Brothers Medical Publishers (P) Ltd.
4838/24, Ansari Road, Daryaganj
New Delhi 110 002, India
Phone: +91-11-43574357
Fax: +91-11-43574314
E-mail: jaypee@jaypeebrothers.com

Overseas Office
JP Medical Ltd.
83, Victoria Street, London
SW1H 0HW (UK)
Phone: +44-20 3170 8910
Fax: +44(0)20 3008 6180
E-mail: info@jpmedpub.com

Website: www.jaypeebrothers.com
Website: www.jaypeedigital.com

Inquiries for bulk sales may be solicited at: jaypee@jaypeebrothers.com

Mental Health Nursing Practical Record Book for General Nursing and Midwifery

First Edition: 2016

Reprint: **2024**

ISBN 978-93-86056-81-8

Printed at: Sterling Graphics Pvt. Ltd.

Preface

Mental health nurses work with people suffering from various mental health conditions and also with their caregivers. The work involves in helping the patients in not only recovering from their illness, but also come to terms in order to lead a positive life. They often work in multidisciplinary teams, liaising with psychiatrists, psychologists, occupational therapists, social workers and other health professionals.

As a mental health nurse, he/she is required to deal with acute and chronic patients in a variety of settings, which may range from community healthcare centers to hospital outpatient and inpatient departments. In order to play his/her varied role in an effective manner, it is imperative that the mental health nurse is both knowledgable and competent. Towards achieving this end, the nurse is required to gain expertise in both theoretical and clinical areas.

During my teaching experience, both at undergraduate and graduate levels, I observed that the students are submitting their assignments in loose sheets and later collating them, thus giving a muddled appearance. Finally, the nursing students do not have any standard formats to look to, resulting in compiling the information in a haphazard manner and also omitting the basic information in certain instances. This practical record book has been designed with the basic idea to redress such issues.

There has been a genuine effort on my part to design the record in such a way as to help the student document the necessary information in a systematic and scientific manner. It not only includes the outline of various assignments to be completed by the students during their psychiatric clinical experience postings, but also fulfill the clinical experience as prescribed by INC syllabus. Notes on a few topics have also been provided at the beginning to assist the student nurses.

I sincerely hope that this publication will help the student nurses achieve essential skills and also the desired results in their examinations.

R Sreevani

CLINICAL EXPERIENCE RECORD OF MENTAL HEALTH NURSING

Photograph

Name of the student : ....

Register No. : ....

Year : ....

Name and address of the institution : ....

....

....

....

Name of the hospital/nursing home (where the mental health nursing clinical practice attended) : ....

....

....

....

Signature of Student	Signature of Class Coordinator	Signature of Principal
Date:	Date:	Date:

CLINICAL REQUIREMENTS FOR 2nd YEAR GENERAL NURSING AND MIDWIFERY AS PER INDIAN NURSING COUNCIL, NEW DELHI, INDIA

Area	Nursing Procedure	Recommended	Completed
Psychiatric OPD	1. Objectives, philosophy and physical setup of the mental hospital / nursing home / institution	1	
	2. History taking	1	
	3. Mental status examination	2	
	4. Observational report of OPD	1	
Child Guidance Clinic	5. History taking	1	
	6. Mental status examination	1	
	7. Health education	1	
	8. Observational report of child guidance clinic	1	
Inpatient Ward	9. Admission procedure	1	
	10. Discharge procedure	1	
	11. History taking	1	
	12. Mental status examination	2	
	13. Process recording	2	
	14. Care plan	1	
	15. Case study	1	
	16. Case presentation	1	
	17. Assist the patient for electroconvulsive therapy	1	
	18. Assist the patient for psychotherapy	1	
	19. Health education	1	
	20. Drug book	1	

Signature of Student

This is to certify that he/she has completed clinical requirements as per the syllabus.

Signature of Student
Date:

Signature of Class Coordinator
Date:

Signature of Principal
Date:

Signature of Internal Examiner
Date:

Signature of External Examiner
Date:

Contents

Part I
GENERAL INFORMATION

SHORT NOTES ON NURSING PROCESS IN PSYCHIATRIC NURSING

DEFINITION

"Nursing process is an orderly, systematic manner of determining the patient's problems, making plans to solve them, initiating the plan or assigning others to implement it and evaluating the extent to which the plan was effective in resolving the problems identified".

–Yura and Walsh, 1978

The steps in nursing process supply an organized approach for providing quality psychiatric mental health nursing care. The five steps involved are the same as those used in other nursing specialties, such as medical-surgical nursing, maternity nursing, pediatric nursing. Differences for this specialty, however exist in terms of the manner and focus of the nurse's observations, the particulars of interviewing during data collection and the types of interventions used for identifying problems.

The five steps in nursing process are (Fig. 1.1):

1. Assessment or gathering data.
2. Diagnosis or identifying a problem.
3. Planning or creating a plan to achieve desired outcomes.
4. Implementation or enacting the plan.
5. Evaluation or determining the effectiveness of the plan.

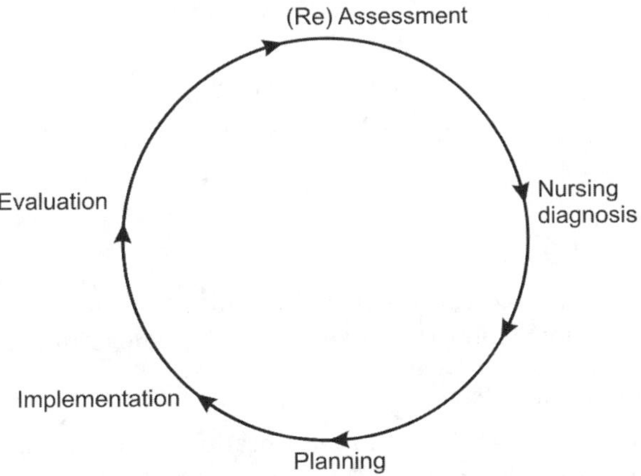

Fig. 1.1: Steps in nursing process

NURSING ASSESSMENT

Assessment involves the collection, organization and analysis of information about the patient's health. In psychiatric mental health nursing, this process is often referred to as a psychosocial assessment. The nurse obtains assessment data from several sources (Box 1.1).

Box 1.1: Components of Psychosocial Assessment

- Interview with the patient and his family members
- History and physical examination
- Mental status examination
- Records from other health care facilities or prior treatment
- Laboratory and psychological tests
- Assessment by other professionals and paraprofessionals

1. Clinical Interview

The interview allows the nurse to hear the patient's perspective on the problem (Box 1.2).

Box 1.2: Effective Interview Skills

- Conduct the interview in a quiet place, ensure privacy
- Be relaxed and maintain an unhurried posture
- Maintain eye contact with the patient
- Be interested and attentive to what he says
- Pick up verbal and non-verbal cues of distress
- Allow the patient to talk freely without any interruption
- When the patient deviates from the theme or loses his track, guide him to the main theme politely
- Use open-ended questions
- Use active listening
- Do not offer premature conclusions and assurance on the outcome of the treatment

2. History Taking

History taking proceeds through different headings as follows:

a. Identification and demographical details
b. Presenting complaints and duration
c. History of present illness
d. Past psychiatric history
e. Family history
f. Personal history
g. Premorbid personality

a. Identification and Demographical Details

This includes the patient's name, age, sex, religion, address, socioeconomic status, hospital number, marital status, occupation, details of informant and information-relevant or not, adequate or not.

b. Presenting Complaints/Chief Complaints

Here symptoms are listed in a chronological order with their duration. Sometimes, the patient may deny the existence of any symptoms and say that he was forcibly brought to the hospital by his relatives. In such cases, information is collected from his relatives. It is preferable to use the patient's own words verbatim, without translating or interpreting their meaning. For example, sleeplessness – 3 weeks, loss of appetite and hearing voices – 2 weeks.

The mode of onset of the illness may be acute or insidious. The progress may be steady and progressive or diminishing and reappearing periodically or staying the same way throughout. These should also be enquired. Sometimes, the patient will be able to point out some antecedent stressful event referred to as precipitants. The temporal relation of the event with the illness, severity of the stress, the patient's preoccupation with the events and the value attached to the event by him may all give a clue to the presence and nature of the precipitant.

c. History of Present Illness

Under this are recorded the evolution of the patient's symptoms from the time they were first noted till the time of consultation. Details of each symptom should be collected. The patient's history may have to be supplemented with data available from other sources.

It is ideal to use the patient's own words. Look for and also ask for any precipitating factors. An attempt should also be made to identify any possible secondary gain to the patient because of his symptoms.

d. Past Psychiatric History

Enquire whether the patient had any psychiatric illness in the past. If so, its nature, duration, treatment and outcome should be noted down. If treatment was discontinued in the middle enquire the reason for this as well the reason for switching over to other models of therapy.

e. Family History

Enquire about the type and size of family and the general family environment. The presence of psychiatric illness on the paternal or maternal side should routinely be asked. It would be useful to construct a family tree depicting the living members, their age, deceased members and their age at death. Mark whether any of them has or had a similar illness and if known the type of treatment they received and the outcome. Note specifically any history of suicide, mental retardation, epilepsy or any genetically transmittable disorders.

f. Personal History

The personal history includes the developmental, educational, occupational as well as the sexual history of the patient. Developmental history includes details of pregnancy and delivery, developmental milestones, health during childhood and adolescence, neurotic symptoms and occurrence of any significant event (e.g. separation from parents, bereavements, etc. are recorded).

The educational history relates to details regarding the level of performance in school, relationship with peers and teachers, academic achievements and extracurricular activities.

In occupational history, enquiry should be made about the types of work, job satisfaction, whether jobs were changed frequently and if so, the reasons for this, work skills and relationship with colleagues.

Sexual history includes details about sexual development, practices and attitudes towards sex. For marital history, enquire about married life and details about spouse and children.

g. Premorbid Personality

Personality of a patient consists of those habitual attitudes and patterns of behavior which characterize an individual. Personality sometimes changes after the onset of an illness. The nurse has to get a description of the personality before the onset of the illness and aim to build up a picture of the individual, not a type. Enquiry with respect to the following areas has to be made:

- Attitude towards others in social, family and sexual relationship: Ability to trust others, make and sustain relationship, anxious or secure, leader or follower, participation, responsibility, capacity to make decision, dominant or submissive, friendly or emotionally cold, etc. Difficulty in role taking—gender, sexual, familial.
- Attitudes towards self: Egocentric, selfish, indulgent, dramatizing, critical, depreciatory, overconcerned, self-conscious, satisfaction or dissatisfaction with work. Attitude towards health and bodily functions. Attitude towards past achievements and failure, and the future.
- Moral and religious attitudes and standards: Evidence of rigidity or compliance, permissiveness or over conscientiousness, conformity or rebellion. Enquire specifically about religious beliefs. Excessive religiosity.
- Mood: Enquire about stability of mood, mood swings, whether anxious, irritable, worrying or tense. Whether lively or gloomy. Ability to express and control feelings of anger, anxiety or depression.
- Leisure activities and hobbies: Interest in reading, play, music, movies, etc. Enquire about creative ability. Whether leisure time is spent alone or with friends. Is the circle of friends large or small?
- Fantasy life: Enquire about content of daydreams and dreams. Amount of time spent in daydreaming.

- Reaction pattern to stress: Ability to tolerate frustration, losses, disappointments and circumstances arousing anger, anxiety or depression. Evidence for the excessive use of particular defense mechanisms, such as denial, rationalization, projection, etc.

HISTORY TAKING FORMAT IN PSYCHIATRIC NURSING

I. Identification Data

Name: Age: Sex:

Father/Spouse:

Address:

Education: Occupation: Income:

Marital status: Religion:

Informant:

Information: Relevant/not relevant, adequate/not adequate

II. Presenting Chief Complaint

(With duration in chronological order, in patient's own words and informant's own words)

III. History of Present Illness

Duration (days/weeks/months/years):

Mode of onset : Abrupt/acute/subacute/insidious
(<48 h/<1week/1–2 weeks/within a few weeks)

Course : Continuous/episodic/fluctuating/deteriorating/improving/unclear

Intensity : Same/increasing/decreasing

Precipitating factors : Yes/no, if yes, explain

Description of present illness (Chronological description of abnormal behavior, associated problems like suicide, homicide, disruptive behavior; thought content, speech, mood states, abnormal perception, biological functioning, social functioning, occupational functioning, changes in ADLs)

IV. Treatment History

Drugs (name of the drug, dose, route, side effects, if any)

ECT:

Psychotherapy:

Family therapy:

Rehabilitation:

V. Past Psychiatric and Medical History

Number of previous episodes/hospitalization (psychiatric) with onset and course:

Complete or incomplete remission:

Duration of each episode:

Treatment details and its side effects, if any:

Treatment outcome:

Details of any precipitating factors, if present:

Substance use details:

Surgical procedures/accidents/head injury/convulsions/unconsciousness/DM/HTN/CAD/venereal disease/HIV positivity/any other:

VI. Family History

Description (describe each family member briefly—age, education, occupation, health status, relationship with the patient, age at death, mode of death)
Genogram:

VII. Personal History

A. Perinatal History

Antenatal period	:	Maternal infections/exposure to radiation/any other check ups Any complications
Intranatal period	:	Type of delivery—normal/instrumental/cesearean Any complications
Birth	:	Full-term/premature/postmature
Birth cry	:	Immediate/delayed
Birth defects	:	Yes or no, if yes, specify
Postnatal complications	:	Cyanosis/convulsions/jaundice/neonatal infections/any other

B. Childhood History

Primary caregiver :

Feeding : Breast-fed/artificial mode of feeding

Age at weaning :

Developmental milestones : Normal/delayed

Behavior and emotional problems : Thumb sucking/excessive temper tantrums/stuttering/headbanging/body rocking/nail-biting/pica/enuresis/morbid fears/night terrors/somnambulism

Illness during childhood : Specifically for CNS infections/epilepsy/neurotic disorders/malnutrition

C. Educational History

Age at beginning of formal education :

Academic performance (specifically look for learning disability and attention deficit disorders) :

Extracurricular achievements, if any :

Relationships with peers and teachers :

School phobia : yes/no

Look for conduct disorders, e.g truancy/stealing: yes/no

Reason for termination of studies :

D. Play History

Games played (at what stage and with whom) :

Relationships with playmates :

E. Emotional Problems during Adolescence

Running away from home/delinquency/smoking/drug-taking/any other (specify):

F. Puberty

Age at appearance of secondary sexual characteristics:

Anxiety related to puberty changes:

Age at menarche:

Reaction to menarche:

Regularity of cycles, duration of flow:

Abnormalities, if any (menorrhagia, dysmenorrhea, etc.):

G. Obstetrical History

LMP:

Number of children:

Any abnormalities associated with pregnancy, delivery, puerperium:

Termination of pregnancy, if any:

Menopause (including any associated problems):

H. Occupational History

Age at starting work :

Jobs held in chronological order :

Reasons for changes :

Current job satisfaction :

(including relationships with authorities, colleagues, subordinates)

Whether job is appropriate to patient's background:

I. Sexual and Martial History

Genogram (family of procreation—details of spouse and children) :

Type of marriage : Self-choice/arranged

Duration of marriage :

Interpersonal and sexual relations : Satisfactory/unsatisfactory

Extramarital relationship, if any, specify :

J. Premorbid Personality

- Interpersonal relationships : Extrovert/introvert
- Family and social relationships :
- Use of leisure time :
- Predominant mood : Optimistic/pessimistic, stable/fluctuating, cheerful/despondent
- Usual reaction to stressful events :
- Attitude to self and others : Self-appraisal of abilities, achievements and failures
- Attitude to work and responsibility :
- Religious beliefs and moral attitudes :
- Fantasy life (Day dreams) : Frequency and content
- Habits

  Eating pattern : Regular/irregular

  Elimination : Regular/irregular

  Sleep : Regular/irregular

  Use of drugs, tobacco, alcohol :

3. Mental Status Examination

The mental status examination (MSE) is used to determine whether a patient is experiencing abnormalities in thinking and reasoning ability, feelings or behavior. The MSE includes observations and questions in the following categories:

a. General appearance and behavior
b. Speech
c. Thought
d. Mood and affect
e. Perception
f. Cognitive functions.

a. General Appearance and Behavior

Describe patient's appearance and behavior. Is he dressed properly? Assess the patient's sensorium. Is he alert? Drowsy? Stuporous? Comatose? Is he cooperative for the examination? Does he make eye contact with the examiner? What is his level of activity? Is he excited? Retarded? Hyperactive? Restless? Does he have any mannerisms? Gestures? Tics? Involuntary movements?

b. Speech

The manner of speaking and its defects are recorded under speech whereas the content and form of speech are recorded under thought disorders. Does he speak spontaneously or only responding to questions posed to him? Assess the rate, quantity and flow of speech. It is worthwhile to record a sample of speech for later analysis.

c. Thought

Inference about the thought process and its disorders are made from the speech sample or the writing speech sample of the patient. Disorders of form, progression, content and possession may be present. Does the patient have delusions, obsessive ruminations and thought alienation? How does the delusion affect his behavior?

d. Mood and Affect

The patient should be asked about his affective state. Compare the subjective report with what is objectively observed. Is his mood appropriate or not? Congruent or incongruent? Labile? Is the emotional expression blunt? Is the affective expression adequate and appropriate?

e. Perception

Has the patient any perceptual abnormalities like illusions and hallucinations? If hallucinating, what is the type of hallucination and what is his reaction?

f. Cognitive Functions

Is the patient attentive? Can his attention be easily aroused and sustained? How is his concentration? To assess cognitive function some simple tests can be administered. The patient is asked to name the days of the week or names of the months forward and backward. He may be asked to serially subtract 7 or 3 from 100 and tell the numbers.

Is the patient oriented to time, place and other people? Orientation to time involves ability to tell correctly the time of the day, date, week, month, year and other related data. Orientation to a place includes correct information of his whereabouts, how he came to be there and other details. Correct identification of people around him ensures orientation to other people.

Patient's intelligence can be inferred from his conversation and behavior, educational level, vocabulary, ability for abstract thinking and reasoning, general information, etc. Specific tests are used when a more accurate measurement of intelligence is needed. The patient's awareness of his disabilities and readiness for treatment are reflected in insight. Judgment may be inferred from his plans for the future.

MENTAL STATUS EXAMINATION FORMAT

A. General Appearance and Behavior

Appearance: Looking one's age/looks older or younger than his or her age/underweight/overweight/physical deformity

Facial expression: Anxious/blunted/pleasant/fearful

Level of grooming: Normal/shabbily dressed/overdressed/idiosyncratically dressed

Level of cleanliness: Adequate/inadequate/overtly clean

Level of consciousness: Fully conscious and alert/drowsy/stuporous/comatosed

Mode of entry: Came willingly/persuaded/brought using physical force

Behavior: Normal/over friendly/preoccupied/aggressive

Cooperativeness: Normal/more than so/less than so

Eye-to-eye contact: Maintained/difficult/not maintained

Psychomotor activity: Normal/increased/decreased

Rapport: Spontaneous/difficult/not established

Gesturing: Normal/exaggerated/odd

Posturing: Normal posture/catatonic posture/stooped/stiff/guarded

Other movements: Normal/stereotype/tremors/extrapyramidal symptoms/abnormal involuntary movements

Other catatonic phenomena: Automatic obedience/negativism/excessive cooperation/waxy flexibility/echopraxia/echolalia

Conversion and dissociative signs: Pseudoseizures/possession states/any other

Compulsive acts/rituals or habits (e.g. repeated hand washing or nail-biting):

Hallucinatory behavior: Smiling or crying without reason/muttering or talking to self, odd gesturing

B. Speech

Initiation: Spontaneous/speaks when spoken to/minimal/mute

Reaction time (time taken to answer the question): Normal/delayed/shortened/difficult to assess

Rate: Normal/slow/rapid

Productivity: Monosyllabic/elaborate replies/pressured

Volume: Normal/increased (loud)/decreased (soft)

Tone: Normal variation/high pitch/low pitch/monotonous

Relevance: Fully relevant/sometimes off target/irrelevant (answer the question appropriately)

Stream: Normal/circumstantial/tangential/blocking/verbigeration/stereotypies verbal/flight of ideas/clang associations (flow and rhythm of speech)

Coherence: Fully coherent/loosening of associations (incoherent)

Others: Echolalia/perseveration/neologism

Sample of speech (in response to open-ended questions, verbatim in 2 or 3 sentences):

C. Mood and Affect

Subjective:

Objective:

Predominant mood state: Irritable/labile/blunted/anxious/fearful/panic/aggressive /cheerful/depressed

Appropriate (relevance to situation and thought congruent)/inappropriate

D. Thought

Stream (flow of thought): Normal/racy thoughts (pressure of thought)/retarded thinking (poverty of thought)/thought block/muddled or unclear thinking/flight of ideas/clang association/mutism

Form (formal thought disorder): Normal/not understandable/circumstantiality/tangentiality/neologism/word salad/ambivalence/perseveration (specify with a sample of speech)

Content

- Delusions (specify type and give example): persecutory delusions/delusion of reference/delusion of influence or passivity/hypochondracal delusions/delusion of grandeur/nihilistic delusions/delusion of infidelity/delusion of control/bizarre delusions
- Ideas: Worthlessness/helplessness/hopelessness/guilt/hypochondriacal/death wishes (suicidal ideations)
- Thought alienation phenomena: Thought insertion/thought withdrawal/thought broadcasting
- Obsessional/compulsive phenomena: Thoughts/images/ruminations/doubts/impulsive rituals
- Phobias (irrational fears):
- Any preoccupations:

E. Perception

Illusions:

Hallucinations (specify type and give example): Auditory/visual/olfactory/gustatory/tactile

Somatic passivity:

Déjà vu/jamais vu:

Depersonalization/ derealization:

F. Cognitive Function (Neuropsychiatric Assessment)

Consciousness: Conscious/cloudy/comatosed

Orientation:

- Time : Appropriate time/day or night/date/day/month/year
- Place : Kind of place/area/city
- Person: Self/close associates/hospital staff

Attention: Normally aroused/aroused with difficulty
Digit forward
Digit backward

Concentration: Normally sustained/sustained with difficulty/distractible
100–7
40–3
20–1
Names of months (backwards)
Names of weekdays (backwards)

Memory:

- Immediate (same test as for attention):
- Recent: (recent happenings—last meal, visitors, etc.)
  Verbal recall - 3 unrelated objects
  5 unrelated objects or imaginary address of 5 items
- Remote:
  - Personal events:
  - Impersonal events:
  - Illness-related events:

Intelligence:

- General fund of information:
- Arithmetic ability : Mental arithmetic/written sums

Abstraction:

- Normal/concrete
- Interpretation of proverbs (give a proverb and ask the inner meaning, e.g, feathers of a bird flock together/rolling stones gather no mass):
- Similarities between paired objects:
- Dissimilarities between paired objects:

Judgment:

- Personal (future plans): intact/impaired
- Social (perception of the society) : intact/impaired
- Test (present a situation and ask their response to the situation) : intact/impaired

G. Insight

Insight is rated on a 6-point scale from 1 to 6:

1. Complete denial of illness.
2. Slight awareness of being sick.
3. Awareness of being sick attributed it to external or physical factor.
4. Awareness of being sick but due to something unknown in himself.
5. Intellectual insight.
6. True emotional insight.

Diagnostic Formulation

4. Physical Examination

A thorough physical examination should be carried out in all cases. The physical examination should include body system review, neurological status and laboratory tests.

Particular attention is paid to recent head trauma, episodes of hypertension, changes in personality, speech or ability to handle activities of daily living. Also, note for any movement disorders. Available laboratory data are reviewed for any abnormalities and documented. Particular attention is paid to any abnormalities of hepatic or renal function because these systems metabolize or excrete many psychiatric medications. In addition, abnormal white blood cell and electrolyte levels should be noted.

5. Psychological Tests

Psychological tests are another source of data for the nurse to use in planning care for the patient. Commonly used psychological tests are instruments for assessing symptoms.

NURSING DIAGNOSIS

Nursing diagnosis is defined as clinical judgments about individual, family or community responses to actual and potential health problems. Nursing diagnoses are used to describe an individual patient's condition, to prescribe nursing interventions and to delineate the parameters for developing outcome criteria.

A nursing diagnosis statement consists of the problem of patient response and one or more related factors that influence or contribute to the patient's problem or response; signs and symptoms or deficiency characteristics or subjective and objective assessment data that support the nursing diagnosis.

The basic level psychiatric nurse identifies nursing problems by using the nomenclature specified by the North American Nursing Diagnoses Association (NANDA).

A nursing diagnosis describes an existing or high-risk problem and requires a three-part statement.

1. The health problem (problem, 'P')
2. The etiological or contributing factors (etiology, 'E').
3. The defining characteristics (signs and symptoms, 'S').

For example

- High-risk for self-directed violence related to depressed mood, feeling of worthlessness, anger turned inward on the self
- Powerlessness related to dysfunctional grieving process, lifestyle of helplessness, evidenced by feelings of lack of control over life situations, over dependence on others to fulfill needs.

PLANNING

Planning involves setting and prioritizing goals, formulating nursing interventions and developing a care plan in conjunction with the patient based on the nursing diagnoses chosen (Box 1.3).

Box 1.3: Effective Planning

- Specific patient needs
- Consideration of the patient's strengths and weaknesses
- Encouragement of the patient to help set achievable goals and participate in his own care
- Feasible interventions.

Nursing interventions with rationales are selected in the planning phase based on the patient's identified risk factors and defining characteristics. The process of planning includes:

- Collaboration of the nurse with patients, significant others and treatment team members
- Identification of priorities of care
- Critical decisions regarding the use of psychotherapeutic principles and practices (identify the most appropriate nursing intervention)
- Coordination and delegation of responsibilities

In this, the nurse will choose nursing interventions appropriate to an individual's identified problem with specific expected outcomes.

Once the nursing diagnoses are identified, the next step is the prioritization of the problems in the order of importance. Highest priority is given to those problems that are life-threatening. Next in the priority are those problems that are likely to cause destructive changes. Lowest in priority are those issues that are related to normative or developmental experiences. Psychiatric nurses often use Maslow's hierarchy of needs to prioritize nursing diagnosis.

Outcome Identification

Outcomes can be defined as a patient's response to the care received. Outcomes are the end result of the process. Measuring outcomes not only demonstrates clinical effectiveness, but also helps to promote rational clinical decision-making on the part of the nurse. Each outcome must follow certain criteria (Box 1.4).

Box 1.4: Criteria for Effective Outcome Identification

- Relate directly to the nursing diagnosis
- Be measurable, time limited and realistic
- Be stated as a desired patient outcome of nursing care
- Reflect the desires of the patient and his family
- Be stated in a way that the patient and his family can understand.

Diagnosis	Outcome	Intervention
Impaired social interaction (Isolates self from others)	Patient will attend group sessions everyday	Using a contract format explain the role and responsibility of patients

Correct and Incorrect Outcome Statement

Nursing diagnosis	Correct outcome	Incorrect outcome
Anxiety	Verbalizes feeling calm, relaxed, with absence of muscle tension and diaphoresis; practices deep breathing	Exhibits decreased anxiety, engages in stress reduction
Ineffective coping	Makes own decisions to attend groups; seeks staff for interaction	Demonstrates effective coping abilities

IMPLEMENTATION

In the implementation phase, the nurse sets interventions prescribed in the planning phase.

Nursing interventions (also known as nursing orders or nursing prescriptions) are the most powerful pieces of the nursing process. Interventions are selected to achieve patient outcome and to prevent or reduce problems. Implementation serves as a blueprint of plan.

Nursing interventions are classified as independent, interdependent and dependent.

Nursing Intervention in Psychiatric Nursing

Interventions for Biological Dimension

- Self-care activities
- Activity and exercise
- Nutritional intervention
- Hydration intervention
- Thermoregulation intervention
- Pain management
- Medication management

Interventions for Psychological Dimension

- Counseling intervention
- Conflict resolution
- Bibliotherapy
- Reminiscence therapy
- Relaxation intervention
- Behavior therapy
- Cognitive therapy
- Psychoeducation
- Spiritual intervention

Interventions for Social Dimension

- Group intervention
- Family intervention
- Milieu therapy

EVALUATION

Evaluation is the process of determining the value of an intervention. Nurses determine the effectiveness of interventions with particular patients. Nurses evaluate selected interventions by judging the patient's progress towards the outcome set down in the nursing care plan.

OBJECTIVES OF CLINICAL EXPERIENCE

GENERAL OBJECTIVE

By the end of the experience, the student will gain an in-depth knowledge and experience for providing comprehensive care to the patients with mental health problems.

SPECIFIC OBJECTIVES

The student will:

1. Get oriented to the philosophy, objectives and physical setup of the institute.
2. Acquire skill in utilizing therapeutic communication techniques.
3. Assess patients with mental health problems.
4. Assess children with various mental health problems.
5. Observe and assist in various therapies.
6. Demonstrate skills in performing MSE.
7. Plan and implement care for patients with mental health problems.
8. Prepare patients for activities of daily living.
9. Perform admission and discharge procedure in psychiatric wards.
10. Administer psychotropic medications as per guidelines.
11. Counsel and teach patients and families regarding common mental health problems.
12. Get acquainted with interdisciplinary collaborative services in psychiatric setup.
13. Develop ability to record and report regarding mentally ill patients.

Part II
ASSESSMENT IN PSYCHIATRIC OPD

ASSIGNMENT 1: PHILOSOPHY, OBJECTIVES AND PHYSICAL SETUP OF THE MENTAL HOSPITAL/NURSING HOME/INSTITUTION

PHILOSOPHY OF MENTAL HOSPITAL/NURSING HOME

OBJECTIVES OF THE MENTAL HOSPITAL/NURSING HOME

1.
2.
3.
4.
5.

BRIEF HISTORY OF THE MENTAL HOSPITAL/NURSING HOME/INSTITUTION

ASSIGNMENT 2 AND 3: HISTORY TAKING AND MENTAL STATUS EXAMINATION IN PSYCHIATRIC NURSING

I. Identification Data

Name : Age : Sex :

Name of the father/spouse : Education : Occupation :

Income : Marital status : Religion :

Address :

Informant :

Information : Relevant/irrelevant, adequate/inadequate

II. Presenting Chief Complaint

(With duration in chronological order, in patient's and informant's own words)

III. History of Present Illness

Duration (days/weeks/months/years):

Mode of onset :

Course :

Intensity :

Precipitating factors : Yes/no, if yes, explain

Description of present illness (while describing present illness consider chronological description of abnormal behavior, associated problems like suicide, homicide, disruptive behavior; thought content, speech, mood states, abnormal perception, biological functioning, social functioning, occupational functioning, changes in ADLs):

IV. Treatment History

V. Past Psychiatric and Medical History

VI. Family History

Name of the family member	Age	Education	Occupation	Health status	Relationship with the patient	Age at death and mode of death

Genogram (family of origin, three generations) :

VII. Personal History

a. Perinatal History

b. Childhood History

c. Educational History

d. Play History

e. Emotional Problems during Adolescence

f. Puberty

g. Obstetrical History

h. Occupational History

i. Sexual and Marital History

j. Premorbid Personality

MENTAL STATUS EXAMINATION IN PSYCHIATRIC NURSING - I

A. General Appearance and Behavior

Appearance :

Facial expression :

Level of grooming :

Level of cleanliness :

Level of consciousness :

Mode of entry :

Behavior :

Co-operativeness :

Eye-to-eye contact :

Psychomotor activity :

Rapport :

Gesturing :

Posturing :

Other movements :

Other catatonic phenomena :

Conversion and dissociative signs :

Hallucinatory behavior :

B. Speech

Initiation :

Reaction time :

Rate :

Productivity :

Volume :

Tone :

Relevance :

Stream (flow and rhythm of speech) :

Coherence :

Others :

Sample of speech (in response to open-ended questions, verbatim in 2 or 3 sentences):

C. Mood and Affect

Subjective :

Objective :

Predominant mood state :

D. Thought

Stream (flow of thought) :

Form (formal thought disorder) :

Content :

E. Perception

Illusions :

Hallucinations :

Somatic passivity :

Déjà vu/jamais vu :

Depersonalization/derealization :

F. Cognitive Function (Neuropsychiatric Assessment)

Consciousness :

Orientation :

Attention :

Concentration :

Memory

- Immediate :
- Recent :
- Remote :

Intelligence :

Abstraction :

Judgment :

G. Insight

Diagnostic Formulation

Name and Signature of Student

Name and Signature of Supervisor

MENTAL STATUS EXAMINATION IN PSYCHIATRIC NURSING - II

I. Identification Data

Name : Age : Sex :

Name of the father/spouse : Education : Occupation :

Income : Marital status : Religion :

Address :

Informant :

Information : Relevant/irrelevant, adequate/inadequate

II. Presenting Chief Complaint

(With duration in chronological order, in patient's and informant's own words)

MENTAL STATUS EXAMINATION

A. General Appearance and Behavior

Appearance :

Facial expression :

Level of grooming :

Level of cleanliness :

Level of consciousness :

Mode of entry :

Behavior :

Co-operativeness :

Eye-to-eye contact :

Psychomotor activity :

Rapport :

Gesturing :

Posturing :

Other movements :

Other catatonic phenomena :

Conversion and dissociative signs :

Hallucinatory behavior :

B. Speech

Initiation :

Reaction time :

Rate :

Productivity :

Volume :

Tone :

Relevance :

Stream (flow and rhythm of speech) :

Coherence :

Others :

Sample of speech (in response to open-ended questions, verbatim in 2 or 3 sentences):

C. Mood and Affect

Subjective :

Objective :

Predominant mood state :

D. Thought

Stream (flow of thought) :

Form (formal thought disorder) :

Content :

E. Perception

Illusions :

Hallucinations :

Somatic passivity :

Déjà vu/jamais vu :

Depersonalization/derealization :

F. Cognitive Function (Neuropsychiatric Assessment)

Consciousness :

Orientation :

Attention :

Concentration :

Memory

- Immediate :
- Recent :
- Remote :

Intelligence :
Abstraction :
Judgment :

G. Insight

Diagnostic Formulation

Name and Signature of Student

Name and Signature of Supervisor

ASSIGNMENT 4: OBSERVATIONAL REPORT ON OUTPATIENT DEPARTMENT

Duration of Posting from .... to ....

Name of the hospital and address :

Average patients per day :

List common psychiatric conditions which you observed in OPD :

List various services provided in the OPD :

Give a brief account of the learning experiences achieved from the OPD posting :

Describe the physical setup of the OPD :

Name and Signature of the Student

Name and Signature of the Supervisor

Part III
ASSESSMENT IN CHILD GUIDANCE CLINIC

ASSIGNMENT 5 AND 6: HISTORY TAKING AND MENTAL STATUS EXAMINATION IN CHILD PSYCHIATRIC NURSING

I. Demographic Data

Name : Age : Date of birth :

Sex : Address :

Income : Residence : Urban / semi-urban / rural

Hospital no. :

Informant : Mother/father/others

II. Chief Complaints (with duration in brief) :

III. History of Present Illness

Onset of symptoms :

Description of symptoms in chronological order with duration :

Functional impairment :

IV. Family History

Nuclear/non-nuclear :

Consanguineous marriage / non-consanguineous marriage :

History of mental illness / epilepsy / mentally retarded / any other :

Genogram (three generations) :

Family history of mental illness :

Living arrangement of the child :
(with whom and where the child is currently living)

Emotional atmosphere at home :
(parental relationships, communication pattern, relationships between siblings, family rituals)

V. Personal History

Antenatal history :

Perinatal history :

Postnatal history :

Milestones :
(motor, social, language development)

Current development status :

Current schooling :

Habits :

Interest and talents :

Sexual history :

Menarche and puberty status :

VI. Current Functioning

Intelligence : Above average / average / below average

School performance : Above average / average / below average

Self-help : Age appropriate

a. Toilet : Yes / no
b. Dressing : Yes / no
c. Eating : Yes / no
d. Bathing / Washing : Yes / no

VII. Mental Status Examination

General observation :

Rapport :

Attention and concentration :

Activity level :

Speech and language ability :

Mood and affect :

Thought process :

Perceptual disturbances :

VIII. Physical Examination

Vision :

Hearing :

Head circumference :

Height :

Weight :

CNS :

Respiratory system :

Cardiovascular system :

Gastrointestinal system :

Genito urinary system :

Birth marks :

IX. Treatment History Till Date

Summary

ASSIGNMENT 7: HEALTH EDUCATION

Name of the topic :

Group and number :

Place :

Date and time:

Duration of health education :

Name of the student :

Name of the supervisor :

Method of teaching :

AV aids :

General objective :

Specific objectives :

Specific objective	Content	AV aids	Evaluation

Specific objective	Content	AV aids	Evaluation

Specific objective	Content	AV aids	Evaluation

Specific objective	Content	AV aids	Evaluation

References :

Name and Signature of Student

Name and Signature of Supervisor

ASSIGNMENT 8: OBSERVATIONAL REPORT ON CHILD GUIDANCE CLINIC

Date of visit:

Describe philosophy of the child guidance clinic:

List the objectives of clinic :

1.

2.

3.

4.

5.

List various services provided by the clinic :

1.

2.

3.

4.

Draw the organizational structure of the clinic:

Briefly describe the physical setup :

Describe staffing pattern and duty timings of the staff :

Mention admission procedure :

Explain various activities provided in the clinic :

Give a brief account of learning experience achieved from this visit :

Author Query: The two "Nursing Care Plan" on page 76/77 aon Page 78/79 are aligned next to each other already plese verfy

Part IV
ASSIGNMENTS IN INPATIENT WARD

ASSIGNMENT 9: ADMISSION PROCEDURE

Date :

Name : Education : Age :

Occupation and income : Sex : Marital status :

Date of admission : Hospital no. : Diagnosis :

Address :

Nursing interventions given to patient
Type of admission
Mention whether consent was given by patient / family member / any other
Brief description of patient condition

Brief description on preparation of patient unit
Describe the preparation of patient record with all the information like unit, bed number, weight, vital signs, MSE and general condition, etc. and write the admission note with details, such as time of patient arrival to ward, mode of arrival, patient's complaints and any other significant information
Describe the orientation given to the patient regarding physical setup of the ward, hospital policies regarding meal time, ward activities, visiting hours, gate pass, attendant staying with the patient and restrictions in the ward
List the investigations advised, such as urine, blood or any other
List the medications ordered by the psychiatrist with details (dose, route and frequency)

Name and Signature of Student

Name and Signature of Supervisor

ASSIGNMENT 10: DISCHARGE PROCEDURE

Date :

Name :	Education :	Age :
Occupation and income :	Sex :	Marital status :
Date of admission :	Hospital no. :	Diagnosis :

Address :

Nursing interventions given to patient
Type of discharge
Check for physician's discharge order
Assess and describe the patient's health care needs at the time of discharge

Write a note on discharge summary
List the medications prescribed to the patient as ordered by the psychiatrist
Write a note on follow-up visits
Brief description of health education provided to the patient
Summary of nurse's notes

Name and Signature of Student

Name and Signature of Supervisor

ASSIGNMENT 11 AND 12: HISTORY TAKING AND MENTAL STATUS EXAMINATION IN PSYCHIATRIC NURSING

I. Identification Data

Name : Age : Sex :

Name of the father/spouse : Education : Occupation :

Income : Marital status : Religion :

Address :

Informant :

Information : Relevant/irrelevant, adequate/inadequate

II. Presenting Chief Complaint

(With duration in chronological order, in patient's and informant's own words)

III. History of Present Illness

Duration (days/weeks/months/years):

Mode of onset :

Course :

Intensity :

Precipitating factors : Yes/no, if yes, explain

Description of present illness (while describing present illness consider chronological description of abnormal behavior, associated problems like suicide, homicide, disruptive behavior; thought content, speech, mood states, abnormal perception, biological functioning, social functioning, occupational functioning, changes in ADLs):

IV. Treatment History

V. Past Psychiatric and Medical History

VI. Family History

Name of the family member	Age	Education	Occupation	Health status	Relationship with the patient	Age at death and mode of death

Genogram (family of origin, three generations) :

VII. Personal History

a. Perinatal History

b. Childhood History

c. Educational History

d. Play History

e. Emotional Problems during Adolescence

f. Puberty

g. Obstetrical History

h. Occupational History

i. Sexual and Marital History

j. Premorbid Personality

MENTAL STATUS EXAMINATION IN PSYCHIATRIC NURSING - I

A. General Appearance and Behavior

Appearance :

Facial expression :

Level of grooming :

Level of cleanliness :

Level of consciousness :

Mode of entry :

Behavior :

Co-operativeness :

Eye-to-eye contact :

Psychomotor activity :

Rapport :

Gesturing :

Posturing :

Other movements :

Other catatonic phenomena :

Conversion and dissociative signs :

Hallucinatory behavior :

B. Speech

Initiation :

Reaction time :

Rate :

Productivity :

Volume :

Tone :

Relevance :

Stream (flow and rhythm of speech) :

Coherence :

Others :

Sample of speech (in response to open-ended questions, verbatim in 2 or 3 sentences):

C. Mood and Affect

Subjective :

Objective :

Predominant mood state :

D. Thought

Stream (flow of thought) :

Form (formal thought disorder) :

Content :

E. Perception

Illusions :

Hallucinations :

Somatic passivity :

Déjà vu/jamais vu :

Depersonalization/derealization :

F. Cognitive Function (Neuropsychiatric Assessment)

Consciousness :

Orientation :

Attention :

Concentration :

Memory

- Immediate :
- Recent :
- Remote :

Intelligence :

Abstraction :

Judgment :

G. Insight

Diagnostic Formulation

Name and Signature of Student

Name and Signature of Supervisor

MENTAL STATUS EXAMINATION IN PSYCHIATRIC NURSING - II

I. Identification Data

Name : Age : Sex :

Name of the father/spouse : Education : Occupation :

Income : Marital status : Religion :

Address :

Informant :

Information : Relevant/irrelevant, adequate/inadequate

II. Presenting Chief Complaint

(With duration in chronological order, in patient's and informant's own words)

MENTAL STATUS EXAMINATION

A. General Appearance and Behavior

Appearance :

Facial expression :

Level of grooming :

Level of cleanliness :

Level of consciousness :

Mode of entry :

Behavior :

Co-operativeness :

Eye-to-eye contact :

Psychomotor activity :

Rapport :

Gesturing :

Posturing :

Other movements :

Other catatonic phenomena :

Conversion and dissociative signs :

Hallucinatory behavior :

B. Speech

Initiation :

Reaction time :

Rate :

Productivity :

Volume :

Tone :

Relevance :

Stream (flow and rhythm of speech) :

Coherence :

Others :

Sample of speech (in response to open-ended questions, verbatim in 2 or 3 sentences):

C. Mood and Affect

Subjective :

Objective :

Predominant mood state :

D. Thought

Stream (flow of thought) :

Form (formal thought disorder) :

Content :

E. Perception

Illusions :

Hallucinations :

Somatic passivity :

Déjà vu/jamais vu :

Depersonalization/derealization :

F. Cognitive Function (Neuropsychiatric Assessment)

Consciousness :

Orientation :

Attention :

Concentration :

Memory

- Immediate :
- Recent :
- Remote :

Intelligence :

Abstraction :

Judgment :

G. Insight

Diagnostic Formulation

Name and Signature of Student

Name and Signature of Supervisor

ASSIGNMENT 13: PROCESS RECORDING - I AND II

PROCESS RECORDING – I

I. Identification Data

Name : Age : Sex :

Religion : Marital status : Educational status :

Occupation : Income per month : Languages known :

I.P. No : Ward : Diagnosis :

Address :

Date of admission : Date and time of process recording :

II. Brief Summary of the Patient Problem

III. Place of Interaction

IV. Description of the Environment

V. Reason for Selecting the Patient

VI. Objectives

1.

2.

3.

Nurse's response: Verbal and non-verbal	Patient's response: Verbal and non-verbal	Communication technique	Inference

Nurse's response: Verbal and non-verbal	Patient's response: Verbal and non-verbal	Communication technique	Inference

Conclusion—fixing the time and place for the next interview :

List of inferences :

Any special difficulties faced during the inference :

Techniques used to overcome difficulties :

Name and Signature of Student

Name and Signature of Supervisor

PROCESS RECORDING - II

I. Identification Data

Name :
Age :
Sex :
Religion :
Marital status :
Educational status :
Occupation :
Income per month :
Languages known :
I.P. No. :
Ward :
Diagnosis :
Address :
Date of admission :
Date and time of process recording :

II. Brief Summary of the Patient Problem

III. Place of Interaction

IV. Description of the Environment

V. Reason for Selecting the Patient

VI. Objectives

1.

2.

3.

Nurse's response: Verbal and non-verbal	Patient's response: Verbal and non-verbal	Communication technique	Inference

Nurse's response: Verbal and non-verbal	Patient's response: Verbal and non-verbal	Communication technique	Inference

Conclusion—fixing the time and place for the next interview :

List of inferences :

Any special difficulties faced during the inference :

Techniques used to overcome difficulties :

Name and Signature of Student

Name and Signature of Supervisor

ASSIGNMENT 14: NURSING CARE PLAN FOR PATIENT WITH PSYCHIATRIC DISORDER

Identification Data

Name : Age : Sex :

Father/spouse : Address : Education :

Occupation : Income : Marital status :

Religion : Informant :

Information: Relevant/irrelevant, adequate/inadequate

Presenting Chief Complaint

(With duration in chronological order, in patient's own words and informant's own words)

History of Present Illness

Duration :

Mode of onset :

Course :

Intensity :

Precipitating factors :

Description of present illness
(While describing present illness consider chronological description of abnormal behavior, associated problems like suicide, homicide, disruptive behavior; thought content, speech, mood states, abnormal perception, biological functioning, social functioning, occupational functioning, changes in ADLs)

Past Psychiatric and Medical History

Family History

Name of the family member	Age	Education	Occupation	Health status	Relationship with the patient	Age at death and mode of death

Genogram (family of origin, three generations) :

Personal History

a. Perinatal History

b. Childhood History

c. Educational History

d. Play History

e. Emotional Problems during Adolescence

f. Puberty

g. Obstetrical History

h. Occupational History

i. Sexual and Marital History

j. Premorbid Personality

Physical Examination

General examination :

Temperature :

Pulse :

Respiration :

Blood pressure (BP) :

CVS, peripheral pulsations :

Respiratory system :

Gastrointestinal :

Musculoskeletal system :

Lymph nodes :

Breasts :

Pelvic examination :

Any other signs :

Summary :

Investigations

Name of the investigation	Patient value	Normal value	Remarks

Mental Status Examination

A. General Appearance and Behavior

Appearance :

Facial expression :

Level of grooming :

Level of cleanliness :

Level of consciousness :

Mode of entry :

Behavior :

Co-operativeness :

Eye-to-eye contact :

Psychomotor activity :

Rapport :

Gesturing :

Posturing :

Other movements :

Other catatonic phenomena :

Conversion and dissociative signs :

Hallucinatory behavior :

B. Speech

Initiation :

Reaction time :

Rate :

Productivity :

Volume :

Tone :

Relevance :

Stream (flow and rhythm of speech) :

Coherence :

Others :

Sample of speech (in response to open-ended questions, verbatim in 2 or 3 sentences) :

C. Mood and Affect

Subjective :

Objective :

Predominant mood state :

D. Thought

Stream (flow of thought) :

Form (formal thought disorder) :

Content :

E. Perception

Illusions :

Hallucinations :
(Specify type and give example)

Somatic passivity :

Déjà vu/jamais vu :

Depersonalization/derealization :

F. Cognitive Function (Neuropsychiatric Assessment)

Consciousness :

Orientation

Time :

Place :

Person :

Attention

Digit forward :

Digit backward :

Concentration :

Memory

- Immediate :
- Recent :
- Remote :

Intelligence :

Abstraction :

Judgment :

G. Insight

Diagnostic Formulation

Nursing Management

Nursing Assessment

Objective data:

Subjective data:

List of nursing diagnoses:

Nursing Care Plan

Assessment	Nursing diagnosis	Goal/Objective	Intervention

Implementation	Rationale	Evaluation

Nursing Care Plan

Assessment	Nursing diagnosis	Goal/Objective	Intervention

Implementation	Rationale	Evaluation

Medications

Sl. No.	Name of the drug	Dose and route	Mechanism of action	Adverse affects	Nurse's responsibility

Health education :

Conclusion :

Name and Signature of Student

Name and Signature of Supervisor

ASSIGNMENT 15: CASE STUDY

Identification Data

Name : Age : Sex : Father/Spouse :

Address : Education : Occupation : Income :

Marital status : Religion : Informant :

Information: Relevant/irrelevant, adequate/inadequate

Presenting Chief Complaint

(With duration in chronological order, in patient's own words and informant's own words)

History of Present Illness

Duration:

Mode of onset :

Course :

Intensity :

Precipitating factors :

Description of present illness
(While describing present illness consider chronological description of abnormal behavior, associated problems like suicide, homicide, disruptive behavior; thought content, speech, mood states, abnormal perception, biological functioning, social functioning, occupational functioning, changes in ADLs)

Past Psychiatric and Medical History

Family History

Name of the family member	Age	Education	Occupation	Health status	Relationship with the patient	Age at death and mode of death

Genogram (family of origin, three generations) :

Personal History

a. Perinatal History

b. Childhood History

c. Educational History

d. Play History

e. Emotional Problems during Adolescence

f. Puberty

g. Obstetrical History

h. Occupational History

i. Sexual and Marital History

j. Premorbid Personality

Physical Examination

General examination :

Temperature :

Pulse :

Respiration :

Blood pressure (BP) :

CVS, peripheral pulsations :

Respiratory system :

Gastrointestinal :

Musculoskeletal system :

Lymph nodes :

Breasts :

Pelvic examination :

Any other signs :

Summary :

Investigations

Name of the investigation	Patient value	Normal value	Remarks

Mental Status Examination

A. General Appearance and Behavior

Appearance :

Facial expression :

Level of grooming :

Level of cleanliness :

Level of consciousness :

Mode of entry :

Behavior :

Co-operativeness :

Eye-to-eye contact :

Psychomotor activity :

Rapport :

Gesturing :

Posturing :

Other movements :

Other catatonic phenomena :

Conversion and dissociative signs :

Hallucinatory behavior :

B. Speech

Initiation :

Reaction time :

Rate :

Productivity :

Volume :

Tone :

Relevance :

Stream (flow and rhythm of speech) :

Coherence :

Others :

Sample of speech (in response to open-ended questions, verbatim in 2 or 3 sentences) :

C. Mood and Affect

Subjective :

Objective :

Predominant mood state :

D. Thought

Stream (flow of thought) :

Form (formal thought disorder) :

Content :

E. Perception

Illusions :

Hallucinations :
(specify type and give example)

Somatic passivity :

Déjà vu/jamais vu :

Depersonalization/derealization :

F. Cognitive Function (Neuropsychiatric Assessment)

Consciousness :

Orientation

Time :

Place :

Person :

Attention :

Concentration :

Memory
- Immediate :
- Recent :
- Remote :

Intelligence

Abstraction :

Judgment :

G. Insight

Diagnostic Formulation

Book Picture of Disease Condition

Introduction

Definition

Incidence

Etiology

Book picture	Patient picture

Psychopathology

Clinical manifestations

Book picture	Patient picture

Investigations

Book picture	Patient picture

Diagnosis

Treatment (psychopharmacological and psychosocial management)

Book picture	Patient picture

Nursing Management

Nursing Assessment

Objective data :

Subjective data :

List of nursing diagnoses :

Nursing Care Plan

Assessment	Nursing diagnosis	Goal/Objective	Intervention

Implementation	Rationale	Evaluation

Nursing Care Plan

Assessment	Nursing diagnosis	Goal/Objective	Intervention

Implementation	Rationale	Evaluation

Medications

Sl. No.	Name of the drug	Dose and route	Mechanism of action	Adverse affects	Nurse's responsibility

Health education :

Conclusion :

References :

Name and Signature of Student

Name and Signature of Supervisor

ASSIGNMENT 16: CASE PRESENTATION

Lesson Plan of Case Presentation on ....

Name of the student :

Year :

Group :

Size of group :

Venue :

Date and time :

Previous knowledge :

Methods of teaching :

A.V. aids :

General objectives :

Specific objectives :

I. Identification Data

Name : Age : Sex :

Name of the father/spouse : Education : Occupation :

Income : Marital status : Religion :

Address :

Informant :

II. Presenting Chief Complaints

III. History of Present Illness

Duration :

Mode of onset :

Course :

Intensity :

Precipitating factors :

Description of present illness

(While describing present illness consider chronological description of abnormal behavior, associated problems like suicide, homicide, disruptive behavior; thought content, speech, mood states, abnormal perception, biological functioning, social functioning, occupational functioning, changes in ADLs)

Past Psychiatric and Medical History

Family History

Name of the family member	Age	Education	Occupation	Health status	Relationship with the patient	Age at death and mode of death

Genogram (family of origin, three generations) :

Personal History

a. Perinatal History

b. Childhood History

c. Educational History

d. Play History

e. Emotional Problems during Adolescence

f. Puberty

g. Obstetrical History

h. Occupational History

i. Sexual and Marital History

j. Premorbid Personality

Physical Examination

General examination :

Temperature :

Pulse :

Respiration :

Blood pressure (BP) :

CVS, peripheral pulsations :

Respiratory system :

Gastrointestinal :

Musculoskeletal system :

Lymph nodes :

Breasts :

Pelvic examination :

Any other signs :

Summary :

Investigations

Name of the investigation	Patient value	Normal value	Remarks

Mental Status Examination

A. General Appearance and Behavior

Appearance :

Facial expression :

Level of grooming :

Level of cleanliness :

Level of consciousness :

Mode of entry :

Behavior :

Co-operativeness :

Eye-to-eye contact :

Psychomotor activity :

Rapport :

Gesturing :

Posturing :

Other movements :

Other catatonic phenomena :

Conversion and dissociative signs :

Hallucinatory behavior :

B. Speech

Initiation :

Reaction time :

Rate :

Productivity :

Volume :

Tone :

Relevance :

Stream (flow and rhythm of speech) :

Coherence :

Others :

Sample of speech (in response to open-ended questions, verbatim in 2 or 3 sentences) :

C. Mood and Affect

Subjective :

Objective :

Predominant mood state :

D. Thought

Stream (flow of thought) :

Form (formal thought disorder) :

Content :

E. Perception

Illusions :

Hallucinations (specify type and give example) :

Somatic passivity :

Déjà vu/jamais vu :

Depersonalization/derealization :

F. Cognitive Function (Neuropsychiatric Assessment)

Consciousness :

Orientation

Time :

Place :

Person :

Attention :

Concentration :

Memory

- Immediate :

- Recent :
- Remote :

Intelligence :

Abstraction :

Judgment :

G. Insight

Diagnostic Formulation

Book Picture of Disease Condition

Introduction

Definition

Incidence

Etiology

Book picture	Patient picture

Psychopathology

Clinical manifestations

Book picture	Patient picture

Investigations

Book picture	Patient picture

Diagnosis

Treatment (psychopharmacological and psychosocial management)

Book picture	Patient picture

Nursing Management

Nursing Assessment

Objective data:

Subjective data:

List of nursing diagnosis :

Nursing Care Plan

Assessment	Nursing diagnosis	Goal/Objective	Intervention

Implementation	Rationale	Evaluation

Nursing Care Plan

Assessment	Nursing diagnosis	Goal/Objective	Intervention

Implementation	Rationale	Evaluation

Medications

Sl. No.	Name of the drug	Dose and route	Mechanism of action	Adverse affects	Nurse's responsibility

Health education :

Conclusion :

References :

Name and Signature of Student

Name and Signature of Supervisor

ASSIGNMENT 17: ASSIST THE PATIENT FOR ELECTROCONVULSIVE THERAPY

I. Identification Data

Name of the patient : Age : Sex :

Religion : I.P. No. : Marital status :

Education : Occupation : Address :

Informant :

II. Presenting Chief Complaints

III. Brief description of the Patient Illness

IV. Mental Status Examination

General appearance and behavior:

Speech:

Mood:

Thought:

Perception:

Cognitive function:

Insight:

Judgment:

Diagnostic formulation:

V. Physical Examination

VI. Assessment of Patient's and Family's Knowledge of Indications, Side Effects, Therapeutic Effects and Risks Associated with ECT

VII. Pre-ECT Care Checklist

Sl. No.	Particulars	Yes/No
1	Informed consent	
2	Assess vital signs	
3	Nil by mouth (6-8 hrs.)	
4	Withhold night dose of drugs	
5	Withhold oral medications in the morning	
6	Head shampooing	
7	Remove jewels, prosthesis, dentures, contact lens, etc.	
8	Remove tight clothing	
9	Empty bladder and bowel just before ECT	
10	Pre-ECT medications	

VIII. Intra Procedure Care Checklist

Sl. No.	Particulars	Yes/No
1	Place the patient comfortably on the ECT table	
2	Stay with the patient	
3	Insert mouth gag	
4	Apply gel and electrodes	
5	Monitor voltage intensity and duration of electrical activity	
6	Monitor seizure activity	
7	Monitor vital signs	

IX. Post Procedure Care Checklist

Sl. No.	Particulars	Yes/No
1	Place patient in sideline position	
2	Monitor vital signs	
3	Oxygen administration	
4	Assess for postictal confusion	
5	Use of side rails to prevent falls	
6	Re-orient the patient after recovery	
7	Recording the case	

Summary

List the equipments available in ECT room:

List the medications available in ECT room:

Describe the staffing pattern and duty timings of the staff:

Draw and describe the physical layout of the ECT room:

Name and Signature of Student

Name and Signature of Supervisor

ASSIGNMENT 18: ASSIST THE PATIENT FOR PSYCHOTHERAPY

I. Demographic Data

Name of the patient : Age : Sex :

Religion : I.P. No. : Marital status :

Education : Occupation : Address :

Informant :

II. Brief Description of Present Illness

III. Brief Description of Mental Status Examination

IV. Treatment

V. Indications for Psychotherapy

VI. Problems Identified for Workup

VII. Brief Description of Psychotherapy given to the Patient

Session no :

Place :

Time :

Psychotherapy approach :

Techniques used by the therapist :

Plan for next session :

Homeworks, if any (given to the patient) :

Outcome of the session :

Summary

Name and Signature of Student

Name and Signature of Supervisor

ASSIGNMENT 19: HEALTH EDUCATION

Name of the topic :

Group and number :

Place :

Date and time :

Duration of health education :

Name of the student :

Name of the supervisor :

Method of teaching :

AV aids :

General objective :

Specific objectives :

Specific objective	Content	AV aids	Evaluation

Specific objective	Content	AV aids	Evaluation

Specific objective	Content	AV aids	Evaluation

Specific objective	Content	AV aids	Evaluation

References :

Name and Signature of Student

Name and Signature of Supervisor

ASSIGNMENT 20: DRUG BOOK

Pharmacological name and trade name	Dose and route	Mechanism of action	Indications	Contra-indications	Adverse effects	Nurse's responsibility

Pharmacological name and trade name	Dose and route	Mechanism of action	Indications	Contra-indications	Adverse effects	Nurse's responsibility

Pharmacological name and trade name	Dose and route	Mechanism of action	Indications	Contra-indications	Adverse effects	Nurse's responsibility

Pharmacological name and trade name	Dose and route	Mechanism of action	Indications	Contra-indications	Adverse effects	Nurse's responsibility

Pharmacological name and trade name	Dose and route	Mechanism of action	Indications	Contra-indications	Adverse effects	Nurse's responsibility

Pharmacological name and trade name	Dose and route	Mechanism of action	Indications	Contra-indications	Adverse effects	Nurse's responsibility

Pharmacological name and trade name	Dose and route	Mechanism of action	Indications	Contra-indications	Adverse effects	Nurse's responsibility

Pharmacological name and trade name	Dose and route	Mechanism of action	Indications	Contra-indications	Adverse effects	Nurse's responsibility

Pharmacological name and trade name	Dose and route	Mechanism of action	Indications	Contra-indications	Adverse effects	Nurse's responsibility

Pharmacological name and trade name	Dose and route	Mechanism of action	Indications	Contra-indications	Adverse effects	Nurse's responsibility

Pharmacological name and trade name	Dose and route	Mechanism of action	Indications	Contra-indications	Adverse effects	Nurse's responsibility

Pharmacological name and trade name	Dose and route	Mechanism of action	Indications	Contra-indications	Adverse effects	Nurse's responsibility

Pharmacological name and trade name	Dose and route	Mechanism of action	Indications	Contra-indications	Adverse effects	Nurse's responsibility

Pharmacological name and trade name	Dose and route	Mechanism of action	Indications	Contra-indications	Adverse effects	Nurse's responsibility

Pharmacological name and trade name	Dose and route	Mechanism of action	Indications	Contra-indications	Adverse effects	Nurse's responsibility

Pharmacological name and trade name	Dose and route	Mechanism of action	Indications	Contra-indications	Adverse effects	Nurse's responsibility

Pharmacological name and trade name	Dose and route	Mechanism of action	Indications	Contra-indications	Adverse effects	Nurse's responsibility

Pharmacological name and trade name	Dose and route	Mechanism of action	Indications	Contra-indications	Adverse effects	Nurse's responsibility

Pharmacological name and trade name	Dose and route	Mechanism of action	Indications	Contra-indications	Adverse effects	Nurse's responsibility

Pharmacological name and trade name	Dose and route	Mechanism of action	Indications	Contra-indications	Adverse effects	Nurse's responsibility

Part V
EVALUATION OF CLINICAL PERFORMANCE

Name of the student :

Register No :

Period : From .... To ....

Name of the Supervisors Max. Marks: 250

Area	Nursing Procedure	Max. Marks	Marks Obtained
Psychiatric OPD	1. Objectives, philosophy and physical set up of the mental hospital / nursing home / institution	5	
	2. History taking	10	
	3. Mental status examination (2)	20	
	4. Observational report of OPD	5	
Child Guidance Clinic	5. History taking	10	
	6. Mental status examination	10	
	7. Health education	10	
	8. Observational report of child guidance clinic	5	
Inpatient Ward	9. Admission procedure	5	
	10. Discharge procedure	5	
	11. History taking	10	
	12. Mental status examination (2)	20	
	13. Process recording (2)	20	
	14. Care plan	10	
	15. Case study	10	
	16. Case presentation	10	
	17. Assist the patient for electroconvulsive therapy	5	
	18. Assist the patient for psychotherapy	5	
	19. Health education	10	
	20. Drug book	40	
Professional Qualities	21. Communication and interpersonal skills	5	
	22. Punctuality	5	
	23. Professional bearing and grooming	5	
	24. Use of learning opportunities	5	
	25. Sense of responsibilities	5	
	Total	**250**	

Remarks of Supervisors

Signature of Supervisors with date

Signature of Student with date